Thrombotic Thrombocytopenic Purpura (TTP) and Hemolytic Uremic Syndrome (HUS): Fast Focus Study Guide

JT Thomas, MD

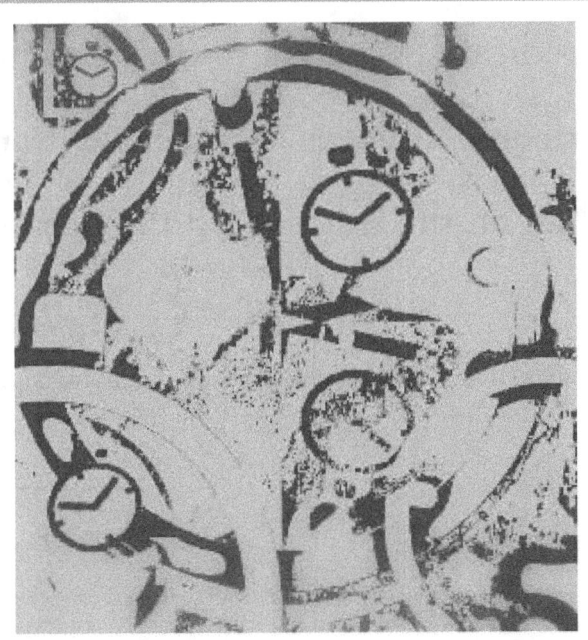

Acknowledgements

I dedicate this book to my beautiful wife and children, who I love more than all the water in all the oceans and all the seas.

CONTENTS

- This book is written to help the reader further understand the Thrombotic Thrombocytopenic Purpura (TTP) and Hemolytic Uremic Syndrome (HUS).

- This book is written in a simple and easy to read format designed for medical students, residents and physicians who are preparing for boards.

- This book simplifies a complicated medical issue so you will remember the important details.

- You will not get caught up in the minutia. Just the facts are found in this book.

- This Fast Focus Study Guide will provide you with a practical review of the key information you need to know.

Thrombotic thrombocytopenic purpura (TTP) is characterized by thrombotic microangiopathies with thrombocytopenia associated with microangiopathic hemolytic anemia.

TTP is an autoimmune disease caused by inhibitory IgG autoantibodies (less frequently, IgM or IgA) directed against the ADAMTS13.

Patients with TTP will have thrombocytopenia (often below <20,000), microangiopathic hemolytic anemia with schistocytes on peripheral smear, elevated LDH and a negative direct coombs (DAT).

TTP symptoms are nonspecific and may include abdominal pain, nausea, vomiting, and weakness. Fever can be present and about 50% of patients will have neurologic abnormalities including seizures and fluctuating focal deficits.

The autoantibodies result in low levels of ADAMTS13.

The ADAMTS 13 is a VWF-cleaving protease that cleaves the Tyr 842-Met 843 peptide bond in VWF to produce the characteristic multimer profile.

The ADAMTS13-mediated VWF cleaving protease is activated to cleave the VWF during secretion of VWF from endothelial cells particularly while free in circulation and during unraveling of VWF at sites of vessel damage.

The ADAMTS 13 protein deficiency limits the protease activity to cleave the VWF proteins resulting in increased ultra-large VWF multimers.

In the absence of ADAMTS13 there is increased concentration of long sticky VWF multimers that accumulate and attach to platelets and causing formation of platelet thrombi.

There will be increased platelet adherence as the VWF multimeric plasma glycoprotein concentrates at the site of vessel damage.

The large VWF proteins will increase platelet adherence therefore causing platelets to adhere and cause microvascular thrombosis in the organs such as the spleen, adrenal glands, heart, kidney, pancreas, and brain.

The classic pentad of TTP is thrombocytopenia, microangiopathic hemolytic anemia, neurological features, fever and renal involvement.

Renal failure and fever are not always present in patients with TTP.

Additionally, about 35% of patients with TTP do not have neurological deficits or dysfunction.

TTP is diagnosed at a rate of 3-4 in 1 million people per year.

There are approximately 1000 new cases of TTP

in the US each year.

The median age at TTP diagnosis is 40 y/o.

TTP is more common in females with a female:male ratio of (2:1).

Prior to the use of pheresis, the mortality rate of TTP was >90%.

The modern mortality rate of acute TTP is estimated at 10–20%.

Even today, the relapse rates range from 10-40%.

Many different possible insults can lead to endothelial injury causing release of von Willebrand factor which can triggering formation of microvascular thrombi.

But most cases of TTP do not have an obvious

etiology.

Medications are thought to cause < 15% of cases of TTP.

Medications implicated in development of TTP include quinine, ticlodipine, simvastatin, trimethoprim, and pegylated interferon.

Pregnancy associated TTP can be difficult to diagnose because pregnancy can also be associated with other forms of microangiopathic processes including pre-eclampsia and HELLP syndrome.

HIV infection can be associated with TTP, thought related to HIV -induced endothelial injury. This occurs more often in advanced disease and initiation HAART is imperative to treating HIV-associated TTP.

Neurological and cardiac symptoms are characteristic of severe disease. It is important to know that approximately 10% of patients will require ventilator support.

Idiopathic TTP will have low ADAMTS13 activity (<10%) and the antibody can be measured. In congenital TTP there will be no antibody detected.

The inherited form of TTP can have variable severity. Some will have symptoms at a young age and some congenital TTP patients won't present until adulthood in the setting of exacerbating factors such as pregnancy.

The only subgroup of TTP with ADAMTS13 activity that is typically <10% is pancreatitis-associated TTP.

Daily plasmaphereis (also known as plasma exchange) is the standard treatment for TTP.

Patients with suspected TTP should be started on plasmapharesis as soon as possible.

If there is an unavoidable delay in plasmapheresis related to a delayed transfer to another hospital where the service is available, then methyl prednisolone and plasma infusions should be initiated.

Plasmapheresis is the most important treatment because it not only replaces plasma containing the missing enzyme, it also removes the anti-ADAMTS13 IgG antibody. High dose steroids should be considered in conjunction with the plasmapheresis.

In the absence of life threatening bleeding, platelet transfusions should be avoided because it is associated with an increased risk of thrombotic events.

If the patient has severe TTP or there is progression of symptoms while on daily plasmapheresis, then twice daily plasmapheresis can be performed or increased plasma volumes can be exchanged.

Low levels of ADAMTS13 is associated with high risk of early relapse but it is not predictive of a poor response to plasma exchange.

The immunosuppressive therapy could be intensified if the plasmapheresis is not having the desired effect. Cyclosporin and Rituximab is can also be used.

Patients with HIV associated TTP should also be treated with highly active anti-retroviral therapy.

A phase II trial of Rituximab for treatment of acute TTP showed a reduction in plasmapheresis requirements.

Rituximab takes about 10 days to begin working in the treatment of acute TTP. The sooner the Rituximab is started, the sooner it will start working. Rituximab has been shown to reduce number of plasmapheresis treatments and result in a faster response.

Rituximab also reduced relapse rates. When patients do relapse, the Rituximab antibody extended the median time to relapse to 24 months.

TTP relapse is defined as the recurrence of acute TTP symptoms within 30 days of achieving remission. Relapse occurs in 20%-50% of cases. There is an increased risk of relapse in patients who have low plasma ADAMTS13 activity (< 10%) or the persistence of anti-ADAMTS13 antibodies.

About 40% of patients who achieve clinical remission but have < 5% ADAMTS13 will relapse. This is compared to 5% relapse rate in patients who have ADAMTS13 activity > 15%.

ADAMTS13 is used as a surrogate marker of relapse.

Hemolytic uremic syndrome (HUS) presents with a triad of microangiopathic hemolytic anemia, thrombocytopenia and acute renal failure. Classic HUS is caused by Shiga toxin producing E coli. Incidence of HUS is increased during summer and early fall HUS is common in all races but very rare in black patients. The vast majority of individual are children. HUS typically presents with diarrhea with or without vomiting, irritability, bloody diarrhea, oliguria and hematuria.

Hemolytic uremic syndrome (HUS) presents with a triad of microangiopathic hemolytic anemia, thrombocytopenia and acute renal failure.

HUS is caused by a strain of the toxin producing E. coli bacteria called E. coli O157:H7.

The vast majority of cases occur children and are characterized by diarrhea with or without vomiting, irritability, bloody diarrhea, oliguria and hematuria.

The most common cause of HUS is infection, however it can also be associated with pregnancy, oral contraceptives, congenital defects in cobalamin metabolism, and can have an autosomal recessive or dominant inheritance.

There is a category of HUS known as atypical HUS that make up about 10% of HUS in children. Although infections can precede atypical HUS, the diarrhea is usually not present.

Patients with thrombocytopenia and microangiopathic hemolytic anemia in the setting of acute anuric/oliguric renal failure requiring dialysis, with no obvious underlying cause should be evaluated for atypical HUS requiring plasmapharesis.

Atypical hemolytic uremic syndrome may have a normal ADAMTS13 at presentation or it can be slightly reduced to a range of about 30–40%.

Atypical HUS is caused by dysregulation of the complement system associated with gain or loss of function mutations of the alternative pathway.

Complement inhibition is an approved treatment of atypical HUS by reducing the excessive activation of the alternative pathway of complement which is the mechanism of disease in most patients with atypical HUS.

Eculizumab is a complement inhibitor used for the treatment of paroxysmal nocturnal haemoglobinuria. In trials, eculizumab is an effective treatment for atypical HUS in patients who were either resistant to plasmapharesis or reliant on plasmapheresis to maintain remission.

Eculizumab works as a monoclonal antibody
to human C5.

The US Food and Drug Administration (FDA) has approved the use of eculizumab for the treatment of atypical HUS.

Mutations in the DGKE gene that codes for diacylglycerol kinase epsilon (DKGE) was found in some young children who presented with atypical HUS. DGKE is a lipid kinase that catalyzes the conversion of diacylglycerol to phosphatidic acid. When not functional or deficient, there is increased protein kinase C activity that results in a microangiopathic process.

Patients with familial atypical HUS have a poor prognosis, with end-stage renal disease or death in 50% to 80% of patients.

Sporadic atypical HUS may be caused by conditions such as infection, cancer, chemotherapy, pregnancy, systemic lupus, organ transplantation, as well as medications including cyclosporine and ticlopidine.

This concludes Thrombotic Thrombocytopenic Purpura (TTP) and Hemolytic Uremic Syndrome (HUS): Fast Focus Study Guide: Fast Focus Study Guide

Search Amazon Kindle books to find other study guides written by

JT Thomas, MD

Internal Medicine Study Guide

Hematology Study Guide

Medical Oncology Study Guide

Cardiology Study Guide

Multiple Myeloma Study Guide

Differential Diagnosis Study Guide

Rheumatology Study Guide

Cancer Study Guide